SCIENCE

OF

VITAMIN K

EVERYTHING YOU NEED TO KNOW ABOUT VITAMIN K

LA FONCEUR

Eb

emerald books

CONTENTS

INTRODUCTION

The term "vitamin" is often thrown around. While we may have some knowledge regarding vitamins, do we really know all about vitamins? While we may have some vitamin knowledge, our awareness is often limited to what we hear from health advocates or simply dietary supplement manufacturing companies. You may come across countless articles promoting the benefits of vitamins, and they often conclude with recommendations for specific supplements.

The aim of scientific discoveries is not to substitute natural food with artificial or genetically modified food. Instead, the goal is to comprehend what is necessary for a healthy and ailment-free life and modify our lifestyle and dietary habits accordingly. However, rather than making these changes, we often opt for shortcuts and rely on supplements. This is mainly due to the influence of advertising and the pharmaceutical industry. Nowadays, you can find supplements for almost everything on the market.

There are many misleading approaches available in the market. It is important to have accurate information because half-baked knowledge can be more harmful than no knowledge at all. Vitamin supplements may be beneficial, they are not regulated by the FDA, and overdose is common and dangerous. Unless your doctor has prescribed a supplement for a medical condition or deficiency, it is best to rely on whole foods to meet your nutrient needs.

Vitamins have been known to affect your health in numerous ways, some of which are yet to be fully discovered. This is why relying on vitamin supplements may not provide the same results that can be effortlessly obtained through natural sources. If you're not focusing on getting your necessary vitamins from food, you're missing out on a lot of potential health benefits.

You will get all the answers about fat-soluble vitamin K in the *The Science of Vitamin K* book. Learn about vitamin K crucial role in maintaining good health and the latest scientific findings and how these can affect your vitamin decisions. Clear up common vitamin K related dilemmas, such as how to tell if you're deficient in vitamin K and when to get tested.

Learn about the advantages of combining vitamin K with other vitamins and foods for optimal health benefits, as well as the potential consequences of taking certain vitamin K with particular foods or medications. This guide covers both beneficial and harmful combinations of vitamin K, as well as the advantages and drawbacks of vitamin K supplement.

Furthermore, learn about nutrient-rich vegetarian options that are high in vitamin K. By consuming these foods, you can avoid vitamin K deficiencies and maintain good overall health, reducing the likelihood of infections and chronic illnesses such as cancer, diabetes, high blood pressure, and cognitive decline. Plus, explore some nutritious and easy-to-cook vegetarian recipes that can be included in your diet to maximize the health benefits of vitamin K.

CHAPTER 1

BASICS OF VITAMINS

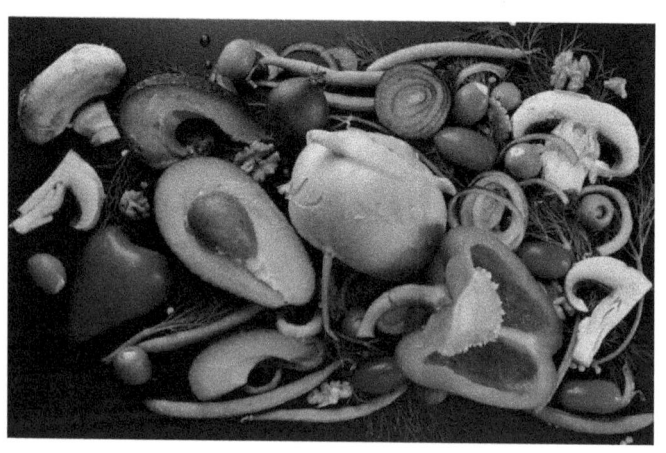

Vitamins are organic compounds required by the body in small quantities to perform various normal functions Vitamins can be essential or non-essential. Essential nutrients are crucial for the normal function of the body, and the body cannot produce them, so they must be obtained through food.

Vitamins differ from macronutrients such as carbohydrates, proteins, and fats because they do not provide energy and are required in smaller quantities. They are called micronutrients because they are needed in small amounts, but this does not make them any less important than macronutrients.

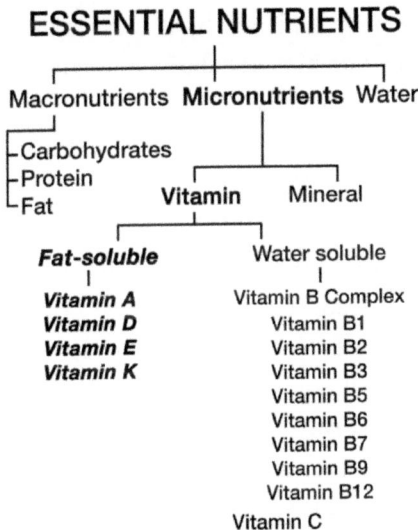

While vitamins are now a topic of general discussion, it may surprise you that they were discovered not so long ago. In fact, all known vitamins were identified during the period between 1912 and 1948.

CLASSIFICATION OF ESSENTIAL VITAMINS

There are 13 essential vitamins that are classified as water-soluble vitamins and fat-soluble vitamins.

Water-Soluble Vitamins

Water-soluble Vitamins are Vitamin B1, B2, B3, B5, B6, B7, B9, B12 and Vitamin C. These vitamins are called water-soluble as they dissolve in water. There are nine of them, including Vitamin B1 to B12 and Vitamin C. Since they dissolve in water, they are easily absorbed, and any excess is excreted in urine quickly without being stored in the body. This is why it is essential to consume water-soluble vitamins regularly to maintain adequate levels.

Fat-Soluble Vitamins

Fat-soluble vitamins are Vitamin A, Vitamin D, Vitamin E and Vitamin K. Fat-soluble vitamins are not soluble in water but instead, dissolve in fats. There are five vitamins that are classified as fat-soluble vitamins - vitamins A, D, E, and K, and these are absorbed by the body in a similar way to dietary fats. When you consume fat-soluble vitamins with healthy fats, their absorption in the intestine increases. Unlike water-soluble vitamins, fat-soluble vitamins are stored in the body and can be used whenever the body requires them. The body stores fat-soluble vitamins in the liver, muscles, and fatty tissue (adipocytes). This means that a continuous supply of fat-soluble vitamins is not necessary, as they are not excreted from the body as quickly as water-soluble vitamins. However, consuming adequate amounts is important to reach the daily recommended intake.

Why do I need fat-soluble vitamins?

Your body requires fat-soluble vitamins to carry out vital physiological processes. In their absence, your body becomes weak and vulnerable to infections and chronic diseases. These vitamins are essential for building your immune system and protecting you from diseases, strengthening your bones, boosting your cognitive health, and reducing the risk of cardiovascular diseases. Overall, fat-soluble vitamins are crucial in maintaining your overall well-being and happiness.

Types of Vitamin Deficiency

There are two types of vitamin deficiency:

Primary deficiency

Secondary deficiency

Primary deficiency

Primary deficiency can happen when you do not eat enough foods that are high in vitamins.

Reasons:
- Poor diet.

- Unavailability of a particular vitamin-rich food in that region.

Secondary deficiency

A secondary deficiency can happen when the body cannot properly absorb or use vitamins.

Reasons:
- Poor lifestyle choices such as smoking and drinking alcohol.
- Use of medications that interfere with the absorption of vitamins.
- An underlying disorder that limits the absorption of vitamins.

Are vitamins Anti-inflammatory?

Let's first understand what is inflammation

Is inflammation good or bad?

Both. The process of inflammation is a natural defense mechanism of the body. It is the process by which the immune system identifies and eliminates harmful and foreign bodies, and begins the healing process. there are two types of inflammation, acute inflammation, which lasts for a few days, is helpful in cases where the body experiences injury or harm. For instance, if you have a cut on your finger, your body sends inflammatory cells to the injury site to start the healing process.

Chronic inflammation is a type of inflammation that occurs over a longer period of time and can last for several months or even years. Even when there is no external threat, your body continues to send inflammatory cells, which can create an ongoing and unnecessary inflammatory condition. This can eventually harm healthy tissues in the long run. Chronic inflammation is the primary cause of many chronic diseases, including rheumatoid arthritis, chronic obstructive pulmonary disease (COPD), diabetes, and cancer.

Chronic inflammation can be caused by several factors, including environmental pollutants, auto-immune diseases, infection, and untreated acute inflammation. Lifestyle factors, such as stress, obesity, alcohol consumption, and smoking, can also contribute to inflammation in the body. It is crucial to treat inflammation promptly, as not doing so can result in life-threatening consequences.

All fat-soluble vitamins A, D, E, and K are anti-inflammatory. Each one has a different pathway to reduce inflammation in the body, which will be discussed in detail in their respective chapters.

NON-ESSENTIAL VITAMINS

Non-essential vitamins are the vitamins that the body can make. Most vitamins are essential and cannot be produced by the body, except for vitamins D, K, and B7.

Vitamin K2 is produced in the intestines, but not in sufficient amounts, so a diet rich in vitamin K is still necessary to meet the daily recommended intake.

Although technically non-essential, these vitamins are still considered essential nutrients because they play a crucial role in the normal growth and development of the body.

NON-NUTRIENTS

Certain substances found in food do not provide any calories but may have positive effects on human health. These substances are known as non-nutrients and include fiber, water, and phytochemicals like flavonoids, curcumin, and polyphenols. While early studies suggest that non-nutrients can improve overall health, more research is needed to classify them as nutrients officially.

Some Interesting Facts About Fat-Soluble Vitamins

• Vitamins were discovered and identified between the years 1912 and 1948.

• The fresher the fruits and vegetables, the more vitamins they will contain.

• Different vitamins react differently to heat. Cooking may increase or decrease the vitamin content of the food.

• While Vitamins D and K are classified as essential nutrients, your body has the ability to produce them.

• Consuming fat-soluble vitamins in the morning on an empty stomach does not provide much benefit.

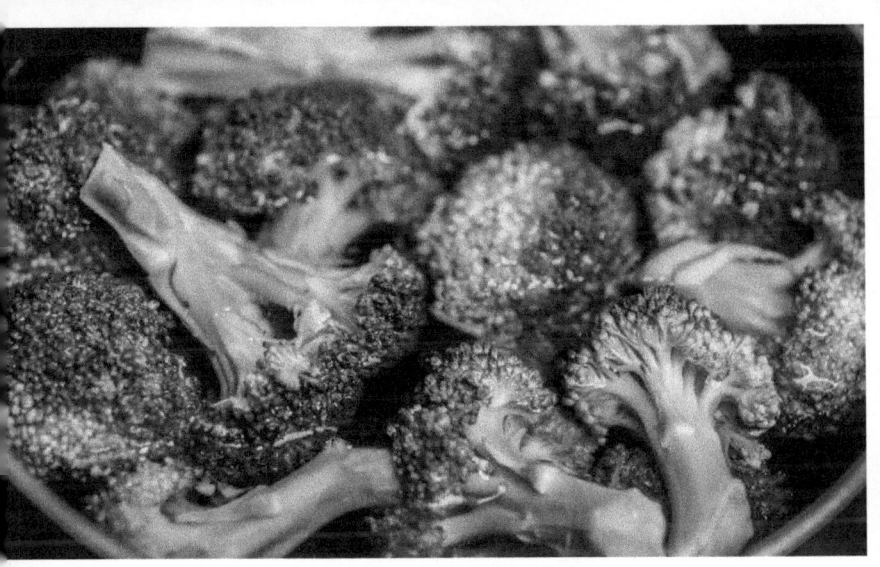

CHAPTER 2

EVERYTHING YOU NEED TO KNOW ABOUT VITAMIN K

Vitamin K is an essential fat-soluble vitamin that your body needs to produce crucial proteins such as prothrombin. This protein plays a vital role in blood clotting and wound healing. Additionally, Vitamin K is crucial for the production of osteocalcin and Matrix Gla-protein, which are necessary for maintaining healthy bones.

Forms of Vitamin K

Vitamin K has two natural forms and one synthetic form

Vitamin K1: Phylloquinone (Natural)

Vitamin K2: Menaquinone (Natural)

Vitamin K3: Menadione (Synthetic)

Vitamin K1 (Phylloquinone)

The primary source of dietary vitamin K is phylloquinone (K1). This essential nutrient is synthesized by plants and is mostly present in green leafy vegetables. Approximately 90% of the total vitamin K in your diet comes from Vitamin K1. The recommended Adequate Intakes (AI) for vitamin K are solely based on phylloquinone.

Vitamin K2 (Menaquinone)

Vitamin K2, or menaquinone, is produced by bacteria and can be found in small amounts in fermented foods, milk, and butter. There are different types of menaquinones, ranging from MK-4 to MK-13, based on the length of their side chain. The most well-researched types of menaquinones are MK-4, MK-7, and MK-9. Interestingly, the body can also convert phylloquinone (K1) into Menaquinone MK-4. Your gut bacteria can produce almost all types of menaquinones, which can fulfill some of the body's vitamin K needs, but not all.

Vitamin K3 (Menadione)

Menadione is a synthetic manmade form of vitamin K. It is converted into menaquinone in the liver and was once used as a dietary supplement. However, it has since been banned by the FDA due to its harmful side effects. These include the destruction of red blood cells (hemolytic anemia) and damage to the liver. Large doses of menadione have also been linked to brain damage. As a result, its use has been discontinued.

How does Vitamin K work in the Body?

When you consume a meal that is rich in vitamin K, the vitamin is absorbed into mixed micelles that consist of bile salts and pancreatic enzymes. These micelles are then absorbed in the small intestine and transported to the liver. Vitamin K1 is transported by triglyceride-rich lipoproteins (TRL), while vitamin K2 is mainly transported by low-density lipoproteins (LDL) to various tissues in the body. Vitamin K is present in many parts of the body, including the liver, brain, bones, heart, and pancreas.

Phylloquinone, the plant form of vitamin K, is not well absorbed by the body. Only 30% to 40% of the total consumption actually remains in the body to provide health benefits. The rest is metabolized and excreted, with 20% leaving through urine and 40% to 50% through feces. This is why Vitamin K toxicity is rare, even with excessive consumption, due to the low absorption rate. However, consuming healthy fats with vitamin K can greatly increase its absorption.

How much Vitamin K do I need?

There isn't sufficient evidence available to establish Recommended Dietary Allowance (RDA) for vitamin K. Therefore, the Food and Nutrition Board (FNB) has established Adequate Intake (AI) to ensure nutritional adequacy in the healthy population.

Age	Male	Female
Birth to 6 months	2.0 mcg	2.0 mcg
7–12 months	2.5 mcg	2.5 mcg
1–3 years	30 mcg	30 mcg
4–8 years	55 mcg	55 mcg
9–13 years	60 mcg	60 mcg
14–18 years	75 mcg	75 mcg
19+ years	120 mcg	90 mcg

Deficiency in Vitamin K

Vitamin K deficiency can lead to excessive bleeding as it is necessary for the formation of blood clots. Although it is rare for a poor diet to cause a deficiency, individuals who take blood-thinning medication like warfarin, those with a disease that affects the absorption of Vitamin K, those who have undergone weight loss surgery, and newborns are at risk of deficiency. Newborns, in particular, require a Vitamin K injection at birth to prevent deficiency. Here are more details:

Vitamin K Shots for Newborns

All newborns must receive vitamin K shots shortly after birth to prevent excessive bleeding, which may result in hemorrhagic disease of the newborn (HDN). According to the Centers for Disease Control and Prevention (CDC), newborns who do not receive the vitamin K shot are 81 times more likely to experience severe bleeding than those who do get the shot.

There are many reasons why newborns are prone to vitamin K deficiency:

- Babies aren't born with enough Vitamin K in their body.
- Vitamin K doesn't cross the placenta well.
- Mother's milk has very low levels of Vitamin K.
- Babies have insufficient gut bacteria to produce vitamin K2.
- The liver of babies is not able to efficiently utilize vitamin K.

Lactating mothers should ensure they consume sufficient amounts of vitamin K through diet or by taking prescribed multivitamins to maintain healthy levels of vitamin K in the baby for up to six months or until the baby obtains it from another source.

While it is uncommon for adults to experience vitamin K deficiency, it is still possible that you may have low levels of this essential nutrient. Signs of a deficiency may include bleeding in different areas of the body or prolonged bleeding after a cut. To address this issue, you can increase your consumption of foods rich in vitamin K. Below are some symptoms that may indicate low levels or deficiency of vitamin K.

Signs and Symptoms of Vitamin K Deficiency

- Nosebleeds
- Bleeding gum
- Easy bruising
- Uncontrolled bleeding from wounds.
- Heavy period flow.
- Bleeding from the gastrointestinal (GI) tract.
- Blood in the urine
- Blood in the stool.
- Blackish stool.

Reasons/Risk Factors for Vitamin K Deficiency

Vitamin K deficiency is not only caused by inadequate intake but also by other risk factors and health conditions.

Long-Term Antibiotic Treatment: Antibiotics are effective in eliminating harmful bacteria, but they can also eliminate vitamin K-synthesizing bacterial flora. Prolonged antibiotic use can lead to a deficiency in vitamin K due to the loss of these bacteria. As a result, it is common for doctors to prescribe multivitamins alongside antibiotics to prevent this deficiency.

Fat Malabsorption: In this condition, fat from your food is not absorbed in your small intestine and passes through your colon unabsorbed, resulting in fatty stools. This can prevent important fat-soluble vitamins, such as vitamin K, from being absorbed by your body, leading to vitamin K deficiency.

Certain Disease Conditions: Certain disease conditions, such as Crohn's disease, can cause fat malabsorption that results in vitamin K deficiency.

Short Bowel Syndrome: A condition that affects people who've had part of the small intestine removed, due to which the body is unable to effectively absorb nutrients from the foods, resulting in vitamin K deficiency.

Liver Disease: People with liver cirrhosis and those with coexisting biliary disease have reduced bile production and bile flow, which leads to a decreased amount of biliary salts. This decreases the absorption of fat-soluble vitamins, including vitamin K.

Anti-Coagulation Medicines: Anticoagulants or anti-clotting drugs, which are commonly known as blood thinners, are vitamin K antagonists that prevent blood clotting. They interfere in the blood clotting process by preventing the formation or working of certain clotting factors. Excessive use of anticoagulants can result in vitamin K deficiency.

How is Vitamin K deficiency diagnosed?

If you experience frequent bruising or excessive bleeding from a cut, or unexpected bleeding, your doctor may ask you to be tested for vitamin K deficiency.

To detect vitamin K deficiency, a prothrombin time (PT) test is used. Prothrombin protein (clotting factor 2) is one of the 13 clotting (coagulation) factors that help blood to clot. This test is the measurement of the time it takes for blood to clot. If the prothrombin time is prolonged, it could indicate low vitamin K levels in the body. To confirm a vitamin K deficiency, oral vitamin K supplements or injections may be administered. If the prothrombin time returns to normal after this treatment, it is confirmed that you have vitamin K deficiency.

Reference range: 11 to 13.5 seconds

This particular blood test is also known as PT/INR or Protime INR. INR stands for international normalized ratio and is derived from the prothrombin time and ensures that the outcome is consistent across different laboratories. The World Health Organization (WHO) has established a method for calculating INR:

INR = Patient PT ÷ Control PT

Note: Under certain conditions, false reports of vitamin K deficiency may occur. Taking blood-thinning medications like warfarin can cause an increase in prothrombin time, which can misleadingly indicate a vitamin K deficiency. To avoid inaccurate results, inform your doctor of any current health conditions and medications before undergoing a vitamin K deficiency test.

Effect of Cooking on Vitamin K1

Vitamin K is relatively heat stable and doesn't get lost during cooking. In fact, cooking green leafy vegetables such as fresh chard and perilla leaf can actually increase their vitamin K concentrations. This is because plants store vitamin K in the chloroplast, and the cooking process breaks down the plant cell wall, which helps in the release of Vitamin K, resulting in a higher concentration of vitamin K in cooked leafy vegetables compared to raw vegetables.

Effect of Exposure to Light on Vitamin K1

While Vitamin K1 (phylloquinone) is unaffected by heat, it is highly sensitive to light and alkaline conditions. It is easily degraded by exposure to light and atmospheric oxygen and can be completely decomposed by alkalis. To keep your vitamin K-rich foods fresh and healthy, it's best to store them in dark-colored bottles to protect them from light.

It is recommended to avoid applying vitamin K to the skin, such as the face and hands, due to its instability in light. Without proper skin protection, exposure to light can cause vitamin K to cause photodegradation and phototoxicity in the skin. This is why the use of Vitamin K in cosmetic products is limited.

CHAPTER 3

IMPORTANCE OF VITAMIN K

FUNCTIONS OF VITAMIN K IN THE BODY

Role in Coagulation

The most important role of vitamin K in the body is its involvement in the blood clotting process. Vitamin K is required for the synthesis of proteins that are involved in blood clotting, such as prothrombin (clotting factor II) and clotting factors VII, IX, and X. Vitamin K acts as a coenzyme, enhancing the action of an enzyme required for the synthesis of these proteins. To form a clot, prothrombin in blood plasma is converted into thrombin by prothrombinase. Thrombin then converts fibrinogen into fibrin, which, together with platelets, creates a blood clot. This process is known as coagulation.

Have you ever noticed a dark brown hard coating on your wound 3-4 days after injury? This is known as blood clotting, a natural process that helps prevent excessive bleeding when you get hurt. Without blood clots, even a simple cut can increase your risk of bleeding to death. Blood clots also play a crucial role in reducing blood loss in situations such as trauma and cardiothoracic surgery. However, Blood clots can be beneficial or harmful, depending on the injury site. For instance, blood clotting at the outer surface of the body aids in stopping blood loss through the cut. But if a blood clot forms inside the body in blood vessels, it can be fatal since they do not dissolve naturally and require proper treatment.

Blood clotting can lead to life-threatening conditions like heart attacks and strokes when it occurs inside blood vessels and obstructs blood flow to vital organs. To prevent this, blood-thinning medications work by blocking the activity of vitamin K and stopping the formation of clots.

Role in Bone Metabolism

The process of bone metabolism involves a continuous cycle of bone growth and resorption. In order to preserve its strength and structure, bone requires constant remodeling. During this process, calcium is released from the bones into the bloodstream to meet other metabolic needs. This allows the bone to alter shape and size. The remodeling process persists throughout the lifetime, with bone reaching its peak mass and dominance by the early 20s. As a result of this continual process, the majority of the skeleton is replaced approximately every decade.

During the remodeling of bones, two types of cells are involved: osteoblasts, which form new bone, and osteoclasts, which break down old bone. As long as the process of bone formation (absorption) is greater than that of bone breakdown (resorption), the healthy bone structure is maintained.

Vitamin K is crucial for bone metabolism as it facilitates the gamma-carboxylation (activation) of several vitamin K-dependent proteins involved in bone health, such as osteocalcin, matrix Gla protein, and protein S. If these proteins are not carboxylated, they remain inactive and cannot contribute to the remodeling process. Additionally, vitamin K regulates the genetic transcription of osteoblastic markers and controls bone reabsorption.

Calcium is a crucial mineral for bone metabolism, and Vitamin K can have a positive impact on its balance. Osteocalcin, a protein, is responsible for transporting calcium from the bloodstream and binding it to the bone matrix, which ultimately increases bone strength and reduces the risk of fractures. However, osteocalcin is initially inactive, and its activation is necessary for it to be able to bind with calcium. For osteocalcin to attract calcium, gamma-carboxylation is essential, allowing it to bind with calcium and concentrate in the bone. Vitamin K plays an important role in activating osteocalcin and preventing the accumulation of calcium on blood vessel walls. This ensures that calcium is deposited in bones rather than in the walls of blood vessels.

Vitamin K insufficiency results in an increase in the concentration of undercarboxylated osteocalcin (ucOC) in blood circulation. As a result, calcium remains in blood circulation and doesn't get concentrated in bone, which results in hip fracture, especially in older people due to bone loss. This is why The Institute of Medicine has increased the dietary reference intakes of vitamin K by approximately 50% from previous recommendations to 90 mcg per day for females and 120 mcg per day for males.

Although vitamin K from natural sources has positive effects on bone health, studies so far have not found any remarkable improvement in bone mineral density with supplements of vitamin K1 and vitamin K2. Therefore, taking vitamin K supplements for bones is not recommended, and any such claims are neither scientifically supported nor authorized by official bodies. To improve bone health, it is recommended to increase the consumption of vitamin K1 and K2-rich foods.

Role in Heart Health

Calcification refers to the accumulation of calcium in body tissues. While calcium is necessary for bone formation, it can also have negative effects. When calcium is deposited abnormally on the walls of blood vessels, it can cause them to become hardened and potentially lead to fatal consequences.

Vitamin K, particularly vitamin K2, plays a crucial role in maintaining a healthy heart. It prevents calcium from depositing on the walls of blood vessels, thereby inhibiting arterial calcification and stiffening. Vitamin K activates a protein called matrix GLA protein (MGP), which is produced by the cells of vascular smooth muscles and acts as a central calcification inhibitor. By preventing the accumulation of calcium salts, vitamin K helps keep the heart healthy.

To get maximum health benefits, it is recommended to consume vitamin K with vitamin D. Consuming vitamin K with vitamin D is more effective for cardiovascular and bone health compared to consuming either alone. This is because these two vitamins work together synergistically. Vitamin D aids in the production of vitamin K-dependent protein, which is essential for proper carboxylation. Additionally, Vitamin D increases calcium absorption in the body and strengthens the bones.

Maintaining sufficient calcium levels in your blood is crucial for many bodily functions. If you don't consume enough calcium, vitamin D will extract calcium from your bones to maintain adequate levels in your blood. This can lead to bone loss and osteoporosis over time. To ensure that calcium is properly deposited in your bones rather than elsewhere in your body, it's important to consume vitamin D through natural sources with vitamin K. Vitamin K helps regulate calcium in your body by activating osteocalcin, which promotes calcium accumulation in your bones, as well as activating matrix GLA protein (MGP), which prevents calcium from depositing in soft tissues like blood vessels.

Role in Cancer Protection

Cancer is the second leading cause of mortality worldwide after heart disease. Many research studies have proved that vitamin K has antitumor effects. High intake of vitamin K is directly linked with lower cancer risks.

All types of vitamin K (vitamin K1, vitamin K2, and vitamin K3) can positively suppress cancer growth and differentiation. Vitamin K inhibits several cancer cell lines by inducing apoptosis and cell cycle arrest of cancer cells at different levels. The cell cycle of cancer cells represents a survival mechanism that allows the tumor cell to repair its damaged DNA. Thus, before DNA repair is complete, vitamin K abolishes the cell cycle checkpoints that cause an apoptosis cascade, leading to cancer cell death.

Out of the three types of vitamin K, vitamin K3 is the most potent but also highly toxic, making it unsuitable for cancer treatment. On the other hand, vitamin K2 has a milder effect than K3 but without any side effects, while vitamin K1 has the least function. Therefore, vitamin K2 is a potential chemotherapeutic candidate for cancer treatment. Vitamin K2 has been found to have anticancer effects against various types of cancer, such as, lung cancer, liver cancer, bile duct cancer, leukemia, pancreatic cancer, ovarian cancer, and colorectal cancer.

When used alone, Vitamin K2 has shown positive results in cancer treatment. However, its effects become even stronger when combined with other chemotherapy drugs. One such drug is Retinoids, which can be used in cancer treatment. The combination of Vitamin K2 and Retinoids has been found to produce synergistic effects. Retinoids work by suppressing the growth of cancer cells, while Vitamin K2 enhances their effectiveness. This combination has also been shown to decrease the recurrence rate of hepatocellular carcinoma (HCC), the most common type of liver cancer.

Another micronutrient, vitamin D3, can reduce the growth of cancer cells by inhibiting cell proliferation and stimulating cell differentiation. However, a potential side effect of vitamin D3 is that it can increase the concentration of calcium in your blood, leading to calcium buildup in your vascular system and increasing the risk of blood clots and stroke. To counteract this, vitamin K2 can regulate calcium deposition and ensure it gets deposited in bone tissue rather than building up in the vascular system. When combined with vitamin D3, vitamin K2 can reduce the risk of calcium buildup and vascular calcification. Additionally, this combination can enhance the induction of cellular differentiation in cancer cells through their synergistic effect.

Health Benefits of Eating Vitamin K

1. Healing a Wound

The consumption of vitamin K, particularly vitamin K1, may enhance the rate of wound healing. In total, thirteen proteins are required for blood clotting, with vitamin K contributing to four of them. By promoting the formation of blood clots, vitamin K prevents excessive bleeding from wounds and speeds up the recovery process.

2. Prevent Fracture Incidence

Studies have shown that vitamin K deficiency can increase the likelihood of fractures. This is because vitamin K plays a crucial role in regulating calcium deposition and ensuring that it is properly deposited in bones rather than circulating in the blood. This helps to maintain bone mineral density and prevent fractures. It is especially important for individuals over 70, as they are more susceptible to bone loss and require higher vitamin K levels to reduce fracture incidents. Therefore, consuming enough vitamin K-rich foods is important to maintain strong and healthy bones.

3. Prevent Osteoporosis

Osteoporosis is a condition that makes your bones weak and easy to break, increasing the risk of fractures. This happens when old bone loss exceeds new bone formation, leading to lower bone mineral density and mass. As bone mass decreases, bones become more vulnerable to fractures. Vitamin K is an essential nutrient for bone health. It effectively reduces fracture rates in people with osteoporosis and increases bone mineral density. Vitamin K activates bone proteins and regulates calcium deposition in bones, which strengthens them. Adding vitamin K-rich foods, calcium, and vitamin D to your diet can reduce the risk of developing osteoporosis.

4. Improve Heart Health

Consuming adequate amounts of Vitamin K2 can effectively reduce the risk of vascular damage. Vitamin K2 activates matrix GLA protein (MGP), which prevents calcium deposition in blood vessel walls. This helps utilize calcium for other essential bodily functions, promoting the health and flexibility of arteries. Increasing your vitamin K intake may help lower the health risks associated with high calcium levels.

5. Prevent Kidney Stone Formation

Excessive calcium intake can result in the formation of kidney stones. Conversely, a deficiency in vitamin K can also increase your likelihood of developing kidney stones. By ensuring an adequate intake of vitamin K, calcium buildup in the kidneys can be prevented. Vitamin K plays a key role in regulating calcium levels in the body and activates matrix GLA protein (MGP), which prevents calcium accumulation in soft tissues, including the kidneys.

6. Boost Cognitive Health

Lower Vitamin K levels have been linked to cognitive dysfunction. Vitamin K is crucial for enhancing cognitive health as it has an anti-apoptotic effect, which means it helps prevent cell death. Research indicates that vitamin K intake can decrease the risk of Alzheimer's disease due to this effect. Additionally, it can reduce inflammation in the brain and spinal cord, improve mitochondrial function, and positively impact conditions like Parkinson's and Multiple Sclerosis. Vitamin K also acts as a co-factor in the synthesis of sphingolipids, which are essential components of brain cell membranes. These lipids play a vital role in regulating cell proliferation, differentiation, and survival.

Research indicates that the use of blood thinning medication can greatly reduce both visual memory and verbal fluency. For those taking medication that acts as a vitamin K antagonist, it is important to maintain a healthy intake of vitamin K through diet, as the use of such medication can result in cognitive decline.

Is there anything I should be aware of?

If you're taking blood-thinning medication, consuming sufficient amounts of vitamin K-rich foods is important. These medications work by inhibiting the activity of vitamin K, which can lead to lower-than-normal levels of this nutrient. Maintaining consistent vitamin K intake can help prevent other health issues that may arise from a deficiency.

INTERACTION

Vitamin K interactions with other drugs:

Anti-Coagulating Medications with Vitamin K

Excessive intake of vitamin K does not cause abnormal blood clotting. There is no known toxicity associated with the intake of either vitamin K1 or vitamin K2. However, if you are at a high risk of developing blood clots and are taking prescribed blood-thinning medications (anticoagulants) to prevent clot formation in organs such as the heart, kidney, lungs, and soft tissue, it is important to maintain a consistent and same amount of vitamin K intake through your diet.

Certain blood-thinning medications, such as warfarin, work by counteracting the effect of vitamin K, which can lead to a deficiency in vitamin K. As Vitamin K has blood clotting effects, it can interfere with the effectiveness of blood thinning medications. If you're taking anticoagulation drugs, sudden changes in your vitamin K intake can have serious consequences. Consuming too much vitamin K can cause blood clots while consuming too little can lead to excessive bleeding. It's recommended that people taking anticoagulants consume a sustained intake of vitamin K through food, meeting current dietary recommendations of 90-120 µg/day. However, it's important to consult your doctor and pharmacist before making any major changes to your vitamin K intake.

Antibiotics and Vitamin K

Antibiotics have two modes of action, either by killing bacteria or by halting their growth. In the process of eliminating harmful bacteria, antibiotics may also eliminate good bacteria that produce vitamin K in the gut. This may result in a decrease in overall vitamin K levels. Some types of antibiotics, such as cephalosporin antibiotics (cefoperazone), are more likely to cause this effect because they not only kill vitamin K-producing bacteria but also hinder the absorption of vitamin K in the body. Vitamin K supplements are often prescribed with cephalosporin antibiotics when these antibiotics are prescribed for more than ten days. However, if the antibiotics are only used for short periods, supplements are not typically necessary.

Anti-Seizure Medications and Vitamin K

Phenytoin is a commonly used anticonvulsant drug to manage various types of seizures. However, it can impede the body's ability to utilize vitamin K by triggering vitamin K metabolism. This may lead to a vitamin K deficiency, which can result in bone loss, osteoporosis, and bleeding incidents. If taken during pregnancy, anticonvulsants like phenytoin may also cause vitamin K deficiency in newborns. Studies have shown that babies born to mothers who took anticonvulsant drugs during pregnancy had lower vitamin K levels in their blood, putting them at risk of bleeding.

Weight-Loss Medications and Vitamin K

Weight-loss drug, orlistat, is a lipase inhibitor that is used in the management of obesity. This drug works by inhibiting gastric and pancreatic lipases, which are responsible for digesting dietary fat. As a result, orlistat decreases the absorption of dietary fat in the body. However, orlistat can also lower the absorption of fat-soluble vitamins, including vitamin K. To prevent any issues, it is common for doctors to prescribe a multivitamin supplement that contains vitamin K with orlistat. If you are taking blood thinners along with orlistat, it may affect your vitamin K status. It is recommended to consult with your doctor and pharmacist to address any potential risk of Vitamin K deficiency.

Olestra and Vitamin K

Olestra is a fat substitute that has been approved by the FDA for use in savory snacks. The Olestra molecule is created from soybean or cottonseed oil and is much larger than regular fat molecules. This makes it impossible for the body to digest and absorb it, resulting in it passing through the body undigested without adding any trans-fat, cholesterol, and calories to your body. FDA has approved its use in potato chips, corn chips, tortillas, crackers, and ready-to-eat popcorn!

Consuming foods containing olestra can lower the absorption of fat-soluble vitamins, including vitamin K. To address this issue, the Food and Drug Administration now requires that food products containing olestra have vitamin K and other fat-soluble vitamins (A, D, and E) added to them. This is to compensate for any potential reduction in absorption caused by olestra's action.

Cholesterol-Lowering Drugs and Vitamin K

Medications that lower cholesterol, such as bile acid sequestrants, work by preventing the absorption of bile acids from the stomach into the bloodstream, which helps lower LDL cholesterol in the body. However, these medications can also decrease the absorption of fat-soluble vitamins like vitamin K, which could cause a deficiency. Examples of bile acid sequestrants include cholestyramine, colesevelam, and colestipol. If you take these medications for a prolonged period, it is important to have your vitamin K levels checked.

CHAPTER 4

10 RICHEST FOOD SOURCES OF VITAMIN K

Here are the top 10 foods that are high in Vitamin K:

1. Mustard Green

Mustard greens are among the richest sources of vitamin K. Cooked mustard greens have more vitamin K than raw ones. 100 gm of cooked mustard greens can provide you with 564% of your daily vitamin K requirement. These greens are incredibly beneficial for your health. They are low in calories, with about 92% water, and are packed with essential nutrients such as vitamins A, C, and E, calcium, and powerful phytonutrients. Consuming mustard greens regularly can improve your eye health, bone health, and brain functions and even reduce your risk of chronic diseases such as autoimmune diseases and heart diseases. Additionally, these greens act as detoxifying agents that help purify your blood and promote healthy skin.

2. Spinach

Spinach is packed with vitamins and minerals. This superfood is high in vitamins K, A, and C and in minerals such as calcium, iron, potassium, and manganese. Half a cup of cooked spinach gives you an incredible 370% of your daily vitamin K requirement, three times the amount you need in a day. Additionally, spinach's anti-inflammatory and antioxidant properties can help protect you from various chronic diseases. Adding spinach to your diet ensures your body's functions run smoothly, and you feel energized and refreshed all day.

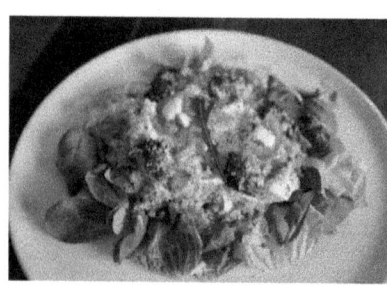

Spinach is packed with essential nutrients that are hard to ignore, even if you aren't fond of its distinctive flavor. It's time to get creative and find some exciting ways to incorporate spinach into your meals. To make it more palatable, add low-fat cream, butter, tomatoes, or lime juice while cooking spinach. Adding lime juice or tomatoes can enhance the absorption of iron while incorporating healthy fats can improve the absorption of fat-soluble vitamins A, E, and K.

Other dark leafy vegetables that are excellent sources of vitamin K are

Cooked collards: Half cup contains 442% of the daily value.

Cooked turnip greens: Half a cup contains 355% of the daily value.

Raw Kale: One cup contains 94% of the daily value.

Lettuce: 100 grams contain 97% of daily value.

3. Broccoli

Broccoli is a cruciferous vegetable that is packed with vitamin K and vitamin C. Half a cup of cooked broccoli gives you 92% of your daily recommended vitamin K. For maximum vitamin K intake, cook broccoli with oils like mustard, 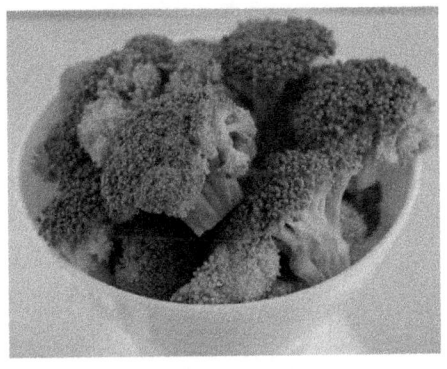 canola, or soybean oil, which are naturally rich in this nutrient. Not only does broccoli help build strong bones due to its high vitamin K and moderate calcium content, but it also contains sulforaphane, which can help prevent osteoporosis. Additionally, pregnant women should eat plenty of broccoli as it is an excellent source of folate, a crucial nutrient for the proper development of the baby's brain and spinal cord. Other cruciferous vegetables like cauliflower, cabbage, or Brussels sprouts are also rich in Vitamin K.

4. Okra/ Lady' Fingers

Do you know that okra, commonly known as lady's fingers, is actually a fruit and not a vegetable? It's packed with essential 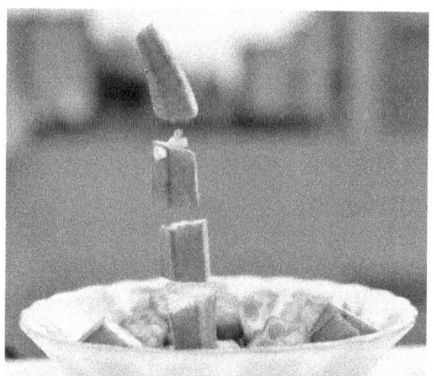 nutrients such as vitamin K, vitamin C, and dietary fiber. One cup of raw okra contains 26% of the daily requirement of vitamin K and is low in calories while providing significant amounts of vitamin B1, B9, magnesium, and calcium. Okra is rich in potent antioxidants, such as polyphenols, which help combat free radicals and prevent heart problems and stroke. It also contains lectin, a type of protein that has anticancer properties and can inhibit cancer cell growth.

For people with diabetes, okra is a great choice due to its high dietary fiber content. Research has found that the viscous soluble dietary fiber in okra can help reduce the absorption of sugar in the intestine, resulting in a gradual release of sugar into the bloodstream preventing a sudden rise in blood sugar levels. However, if you are taking diabetes medication, such as metformin, it's important to limit your consumption of okra as it can decrease the absorption of the medication, making it less effective in controlling blood sugar levels. You should consult with your doctor before adding okra to your diet.

5. Soybean

Soybeans are highly nutritious. They are rich in Vitamin K, Vitamin B, iron, fiber, manganese, and phosphorus. Half a cup of cooked soybeans 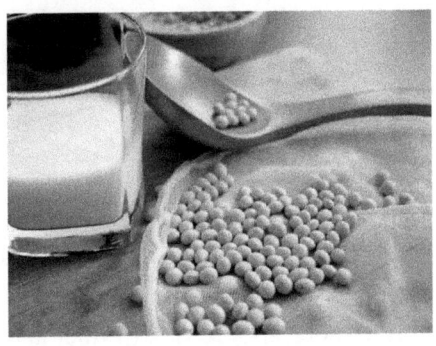 can fulfill 36% of your daily vitamin K requirement, and one tablespoon of soybean oil contains 21% of the daily value of vitamin K. Not only that, but they also contain all nine essential amino acids that your body needs for proper function, making them an excellent source of complete protein. However, to ensure optimal digestion, it's important to soak the soybeans overnight or for at least 8-10 hours before cooking them well in enough water. This is because soybeans contain trypsin inhibitors that can prevent protein digestion and limit the health benefits of the soybeans. Trypsin is an enzyme needed to break down protein, making it easier for the body to absorb. Soaking and cooking the beans properly destroys these inhibitors, allowing better digestion and nutrient absorption.

6. Green Peas

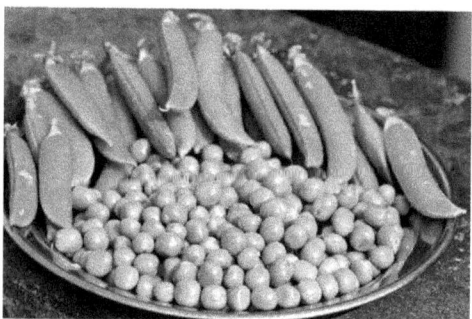

Green peas are an excellent source of various vitamins and minerals. 100 grams of raw green peas provides 24% of your daily recommended intake of vitamin K. These peas also contain decent amounts of vitamins A, B1, B9, and C, as well as essential minerals like manganese, zinc, and iron. Furthermore, they're rich in fiber and protein, which can help you feel full for longer and potentially aid in weight loss. However, it's important to cook green peas thoroughly because raw ones contain antinutrients like lectin, which can cause bloating and digestive issues when consumed in large quantities, and phytic acid, which can reduce the absorption of vital minerals like iron, zinc, and calcium. Cooking green peas reduces the levels of lectin and phytic acid.

7. Sprouted Mung Beans

Sprouted mung beans are a popular choice as compared to other sprouts. When mung beans are sprouted, their nutritional value increases by up to 100%. Sprouted mung beans are rich in vitamins K, C, folate, and iron. Furthermore, sprouted mung beans have more antioxidants and amino acids. A 100-gram serving of raw sprouted mung beans contains 27% of the recommended daily 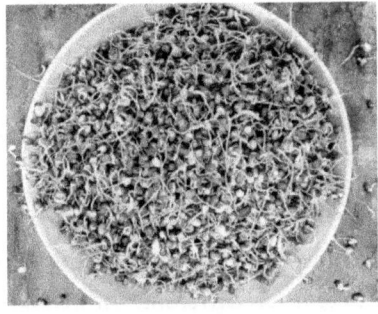 value of vitamin K. It is recommended to sprout mung beans at home instead of buying them from a store, as the latter may be contaminated with bacteria. If you do use store-bought sprouts, it is important to cook them well, as this may reduce the nutritional value, but effectively kill any potential bacteria. For maximum health benefits, it is recommended that you sprout mung beans at home, as this process is simple and does not require specific environmental conditions.

Some other vegetables that can provide you with a good amount of vitamin K include cooked French beans, which contain 25% of the daily value in half a cup, and pumpkin, which has 17% of the daily value in half a cup.

8. Carrot Juice

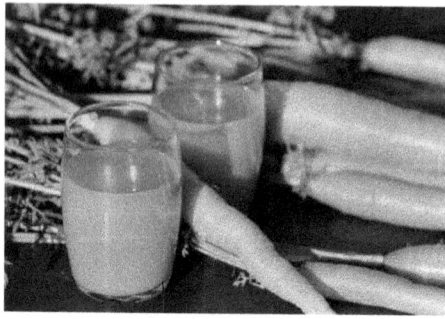

Carrots aren't just a great source of vitamin A, but they're also rich in vitamin K. Drinking just ¾ cup of carrot juice can fulfill 23% of your daily vitamin K requirement. Not only do carrots keep your eyes healthy, but they also provide cardiovascular protection. The high content of different carotenoids in carrots has potent antioxidant effects that can neutralize free radicals, reduce the risk of chronic diseases, and protect against several types of cancer, including stomach, colon, and prostate cancers. If you want to maximize the health benefits of carrots, consider choosing red ones because they contain more lycopene, a powerful antioxidant that can improve heart health, protect your skin from sun damage, improve fertility in young men, and lower the risk of bone, lung, and prostate cancers.

9. Kiwi

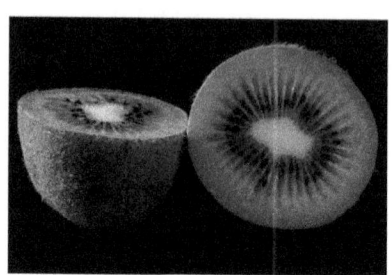

Not just an apple consuming a kiwi daily may also decrease the frequency of doctor visits. Kiwis are an excellent source of vitamin C and provide a moderate amount of vitamins K and E. A single medium-sized kiwi contains 23% of the recommended daily intake of vitamin K. Kiwis are high in fiber, promoting healthy digestion. Studies have shown that consuming kiwis may help with sleep onset, duration, and efficiency for individuals with sleep disturbances. Additionally, kiwis can improve iron absorption in the body and maintain healthy blood cells. Eating a kiwi daily can provide sustained energy throughout the day.

10. Pomegranate

Pomegranates are a highly nutritious fruit. Not only are the arils packed with nutrients, but the peel is equally nutritious. One large pomegranate can provide

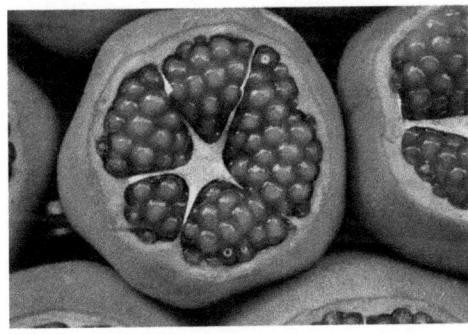

45% of your daily recommended intake of vitamin K. Pomegranates also contain polyphenols, a type of phytochemicals that plants produce to protect themselves against fungi, bacteria, and virus infections. When you eat foods rich in phytochemicals, like pomegranates, they act as antioxidants in your body and have anti-inflammatory effects. The polyphenols in pomegranates help prevent the formation of free radicals, reduce oxidative damage to cells, and decrease inflammation in the body. This can be helpful in protecting against diseases like arthritis, heart disease, and Alzheimer's disease. Pomegranate peel has a high phenolic content and is used in making dietary supplements.

Vitamin K2

Some natural sources of Vitamin K2 (MK-4) include cheddar cheese, mozzarella cheese, milk, yogurt, and miso. While they may not be the most significant sources of vitamin K, it is still important to include them in your diet to meet your body's vitamin K requirements.

CHAPTER 5

POTENTIALLY DANGEROUS VITAMIN K COMBINATIONS YOU SHOULD AVOID

VITAMIN E + VITAMIN K

Vitamin K is important for maintaining bone health, promoting wound healing, and aiding blood clotting. However, when taken with vitamin E, the effects of Vitamin K can be reduced. Vitamin E has blood thinning effects and also increases the metabolism of Vitamin K in the liver, which leads to increased excretion of all forms of vitamin K. While consuming vitamin K-rich foods like spinach and kale with vitamin E-rich foods like nuts or vegetable oil in moderation may not have adverse effects, high intake of vitamin E-rich foods or taking Vitamin E supplements alongside Vitamin K supplements can diminish the benefits of Vitamin K in the body.

VITAMIN A + VITAMIN K

Consuming excessive amounts of Vitamin A can hinder Vitamin K absorption in the body, which is necessary for effective blood clotting. However, consuming vitamin A-rich foods in moderation is unlikely to have a significant impact on Vitamin K absorption, but taking high doses of Vitamin A supplements may significantly decrease the effectiveness of vitamin K.

VITAMIN K + BLOOD THINNERS

Vitamin K interferes with the way anticoagulants like warfarin work. Vitamin K is a coagulant, which means it helps your blood clot, while warfarin is designed to prevent blood clots. Eating foods rich in Vitamin K can make your medication less effective, so limiting your consumption of these foods while on blood thinning drug therapy is important. Additionally, it's important to keep your Vitamin K intake consistent to ensure the effectiveness of your therapy. Avoid eating vitamin K-rich foods within 2 hours of taking your medication. It is recommended to seek advice from your doctor and pharmacist before altering your diet or beginning any medication or vitamin supplements.

VITAMIN K + WATER-SOLUBLE VITAMINS

In order to receive the health benefits of vitamins, they must be properly absorbed. It's not recommended to take fat-soluble vitamin K with water-soluble vitamins (B complex and C) because they are absorbed differently in the body. Combining them may reduce the health benefits you receive from each. Water-soluble vitamins are well absorbed on an empty stomach, while vitamin K requires the presence of fat in the body to be adequately absorbed. To maximize the benefits of each type of vitamin, consume B and C-rich foods in the morning and foods rich vitamin K in the evening. If you take vitamin supplements, take B and C on an empty stomach and take vitamin K in the evening after a meal.

CHAPTER 5

VITAMIN K COMBINATIONS FOR SYNERGISTIC HEALTH BENEFITS

VITAMIN K2 + VITAMIN D

To boost your bone health and cardiovascular health, it is recommended to consume both vitamin K and vitamin D together. These fat-soluble vitamins play an important role in calcium metabolism. When taken together, they are more effective in increasing bone density and reducing the risk of fractures compared to when taken alone. Vitamin D helps increase the concentration of bone proteins such as osteocalcin and Gla protein (BGP), which are responsible for bone formation. However, these proteins remain inactive and require vitamin K to be converted into their active form. Osteocalcin then binds to calcium and helps transport it from the blood to the bones. Without enough vitamin K and vitamin D, calcium may not be absorbed into the bone and instead get deposited in the arteries, affecting bone and cardiovascular health. Vitamin K reduces calcium excretion through urine, while vitamin D increases intestinal calcium absorption and prevents hypocalcemia. Vitamin K2 - MK-4 is effective for bone health, while MK-7 is beneficial for cardiovascular health.

Vitamin D deficiency, along with vitamin K deficiency, increases your risk of hypertension and diabetes. Having both vitamins together can help keep the blood pressure normal. Furthermore, vitamins D and K can improve insulin secretion and beta-cell proliferation in the pancreas, and provide protection against cardiovascular diseases.

For optimal results, it is advisable to obtain vitamins from diet rather than relying on dietary supplements. Overconsumption of vitamin D supplements may even increase the risk of cardiovascular diseases. This is due to the fact that excessive vitamin D intake can cause an increase in vitamin D-dependent proteins, which require vitamin K to activate. Without sufficient vitamin K, these proteins cannot be activated. Therefore, they cannot stimulate bone mineralization or inhibit soft tissue calcification. This can ultimately lead to bone fractures and cardiovascular diseases. If you are taking blood thinners like warfarin (a vitamin K antagonist) while also taking vitamin D supplements, it is crucial to consult your doctor regarding the appropriate dosage of your vitamin D supplements. To get the maximum health benefits, add more vegetables and fermented dairy into your diet for bone and cardiovascular health.

VITAMIN K + CALCIUM

Bone mineral density (BMD) indicates the amount of calcium and other minerals in your bones. When you don't get enough calcium, your BMD can decrease and increase your risk of bone fractures. Calcium is not only important for bones but also for the proper function of muscles and nerves. It acts as factor IV and plays a critical role in blood clotting. However, too much calcium in the body (often caused by high doses of calcium supplements) can be harmful and increase your risk of heart disease. Excess calcium can accumulate in the walls of your blood vessels, blocking the smooth blood flow and leading to heart attacks and strokes.

The amount of vitamin K in the body has a direct impact on calcium levels. If you are low in vitamin K, it can negatively affect your bone metabolism and lead to osteoporosis and fractures. Even with enough calcium in the body, low vitamin K levels can prevent proper utilization of calcium. This can cause calcium deposits in blood vessels instead of bones, which increases the risk of weak bones and heart disease. A combination of calcium and vitamin K is essential for high bone mineral density (BMR) and better heart health. Eating calcium-rich foods like kale and okra, along with vitamin K-rich foods like cheese and fermented foods like natto, can help promote stronger bones and a healthier heart.

CHAPTER 6

DIET PLAN

Here's a 10-day diet plan to include natural sources rich in vitamin K in your diet. Repeat this diet plan every 10 days and you will never be deficient in fat-soluble vitamins.

Day 1: ½ cup of cooked spinach (>100%).

Day 2: 1 cup cooked okra (30%) + 1 cup pomegranate juice (20%) + 1 medium carrot (10%) + ½ cup roasted soybeans (40%).

Day 3: 1 cup iceberg lettuce with Caesar salad dressing (25%) + ½ cup grapes (10%) + 1 cup cooked pumpkin (40%) + 100 g sprouted mung beans (25%).

Day 4: 1 cup cooked soybeans (80%) + ½ cup cooked edamame (20%).

Day 5: 100 g cooked peas (25%).

Day 6: 1 cup cooked broccoli (>100%).

Day 7: ½ cup cooked mustard greens (>100%).

Day 8: ½ cup cooked turnip greens (>100%).

Day 9: ½ cup cooked collards (>100%).

Day 10: 1 cup cooked broccoli (15%) + Vitamin K2 sources.*

* Vegetables and fruits provide vitamin K1, while milk and fermented foods provide vitamin K2, which is equally important. To get Vitamin K2, add curd, buttermilk, butter, cheddar, ricotta and cottage cheese, natto, idli, dosa, and dhokla (and other fermented foods) to your diet.

cheddar, ricotta and cottage cheese, natto, idli, dosa, and dhokla (and other fermented foods) to your diet.

CHAPTER 7

RECIPES

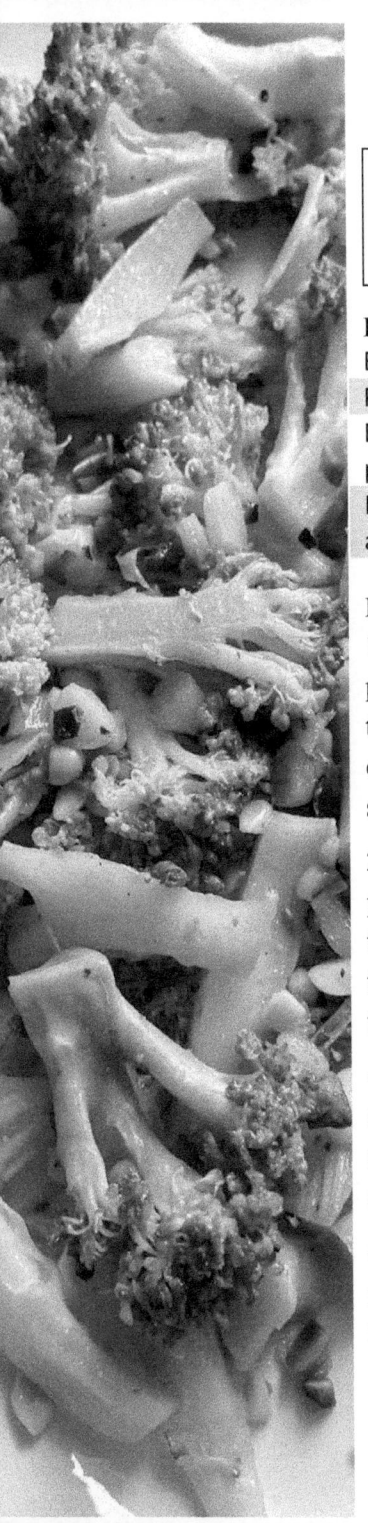

Stir Fried Broccoli

Ingredients

Broccoli: 1	Garlic: 4
Peanuts: 2 tbsp	Salt: To taste
Blackpepper powder: ¼ tsp	Asafetida: ¼ tsp
Red chili flakes: a pinch	Sunflower oil: 1 tbsp

Method

1. Cut the broccoli into 2-inch pieces. Sprinkle salt and steam them in a steamer or pressure cooker, or para boil them in a saucepan.

2. Dry roast the peanuts. Place peanuts in a kitchen towel, cover them with a kitchen towel, and rub them to remove the skin. Crush the peanuts in a mortar.

4. Heat oil and add asafetida and chopped garlic to it. Cook them till they turn golden. Add peanuts and cook for 2 minutes.

6. Add broccoli, black pepper powder and chili flakes. Stir fry for 5 minutes and it's ready to eat.

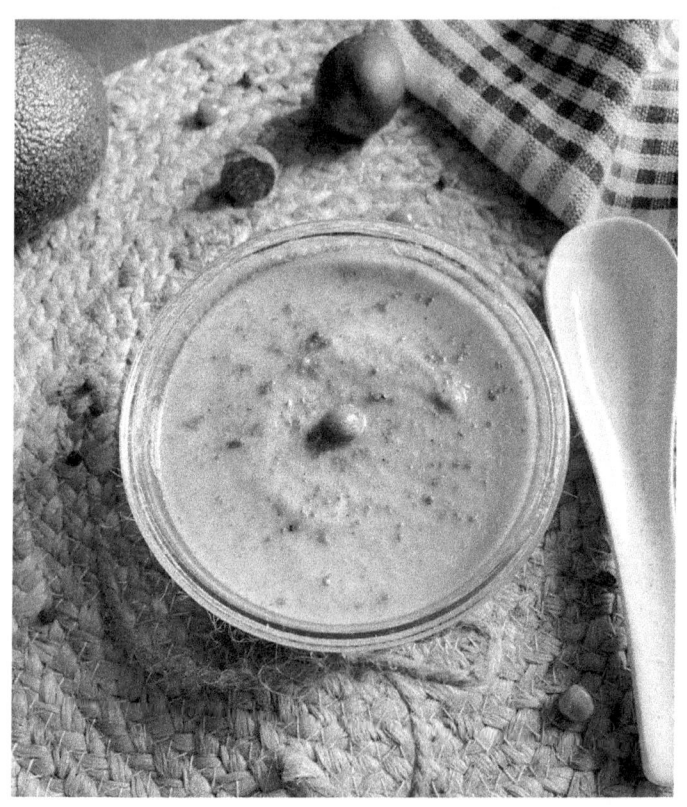

Peas Avocado Soup

Ingredients

Avocado: 1 (170 g)	Peas: 100 g
White onion: 1 medium	Garlic: 5-6 cloves
Cumin seeds: ¼ tsp	Nutmeg: ½ small / ¼ tsp
Garam masala: a pinch / ¼ tsp	Black pepper powder: ¼ tsp
Curd: 2 tsp	Salt: To taste
Rice bran oil: 1 tbsp	Water 400 ml
Optional topping: ¼ tsp tandoori masala	

Method

1. Heat oil in a saucepan. Add cumin seeds. When cumin starts crackling, add garlic and cook for 2 minutes.

2. Add chopped onion and cook till it turns slightly brown.

3. Add fresh peas and salt. Cover and cook till the peas become soft.

4. Lower the flame and add curd. Mix well and cook covered for 2 minutes.

5. Add a pinch of garam masala, black pepper powder and grate about half a small nutmeg. Cover and cook for 2 minutes.

6. Add 200 ml water. Cover and cook for 5 minutes till the water reduces slightly.

7. Add the remaining 200 ml water and cover again and cook for 5 minutes till the water reduces slightly.

8. Take a hand blender and blend the soup to make it thick and smooth.

9. Turn off the flame and add chopped avocado to it. Blend all the ingredients with a hand blender to make a creamy smooth pea avocado soup.

10. Take out the soup in a bowl and optionally sprinkle tandoori masala over it for a tangy taste.

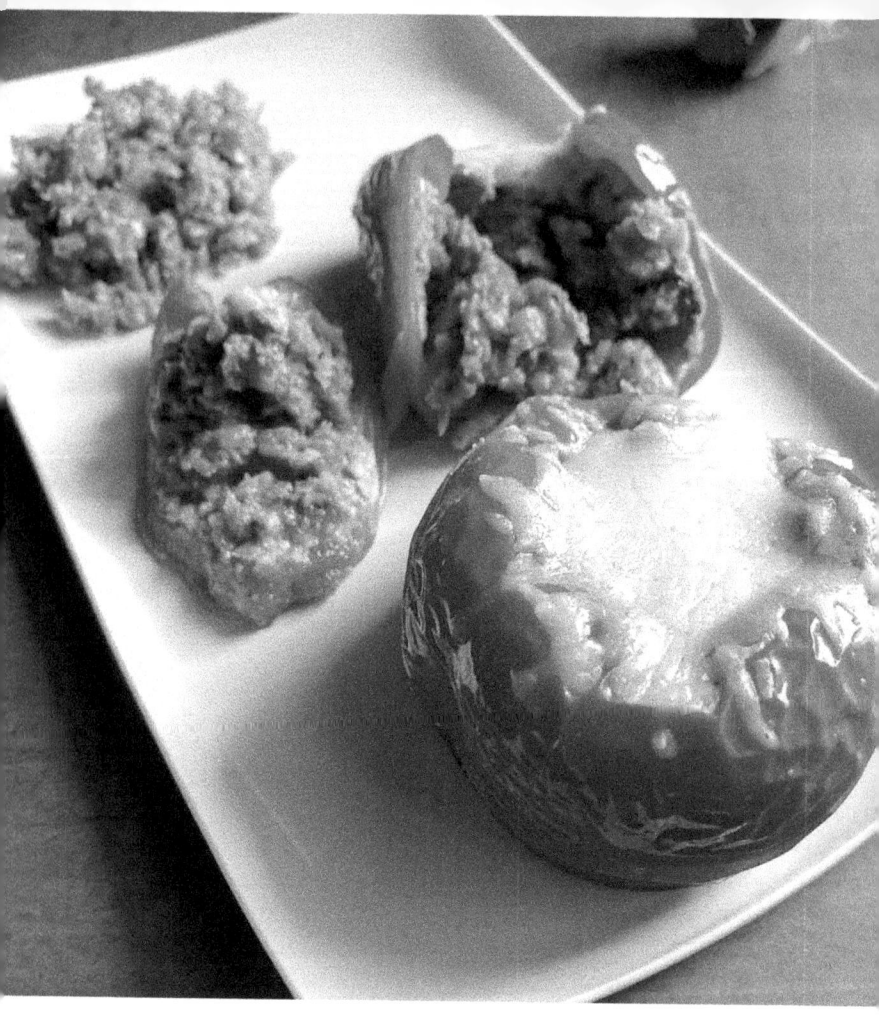

Stuffed Bell Pepper

Ingredients

Red bell pepper: 4

Cheddar cheese: 100 g

Chopped onion: 50 g

Chopped cabbage: 50 g

Cottage cheese: 200 g

Chopped garlic: 2 tbsp

Chopped carrot: 50 g

Chopped tomato: 50 g

Chopped pumpkin: 50 g	Chopped green bell pepper: 50 g
Chopped mushroom: 50 g	Mixed herbs (oregano, parsley, thyme): 1 tbsp
Red chili pepper: ½ tsp	Salt: To taste
Oil: 2 tbsp	

Method

1. Preheat the oven to 190 °C.

2. Heat oil in a pan. Add chopped garlic and cook for 2 minutes. Add onion and cook for 5 minutes.

3. Add all the chopped vegetables one by one and cook until mushrooms and tomato release water.

4. Add salt, red chili pepper, mixed herbs (or your choice of herbs) and mix well.

5. Lastly, add crumbled cottage cheese and cook the stuffing until it becomes slightly dry. Turn off the flame.

6. Remove the tops of the peppers and scoop out the seeds. Grease the outer side of the pepper with oil and sprinkle some salt.

7. Grate some cheese inside the pepper and fill it with the prepared stuffing. Press the stuffing with the fingertip.

8. Place the bell peppers upside down in a baking tray and bake for 25 minutes at 190°C.

9. Remove the peppers and sprinkle a generous amount of cheese on top. Bake again, keeping the cheese side on top for 5 minutes until the cheese is melted.

Sarso ka Saag

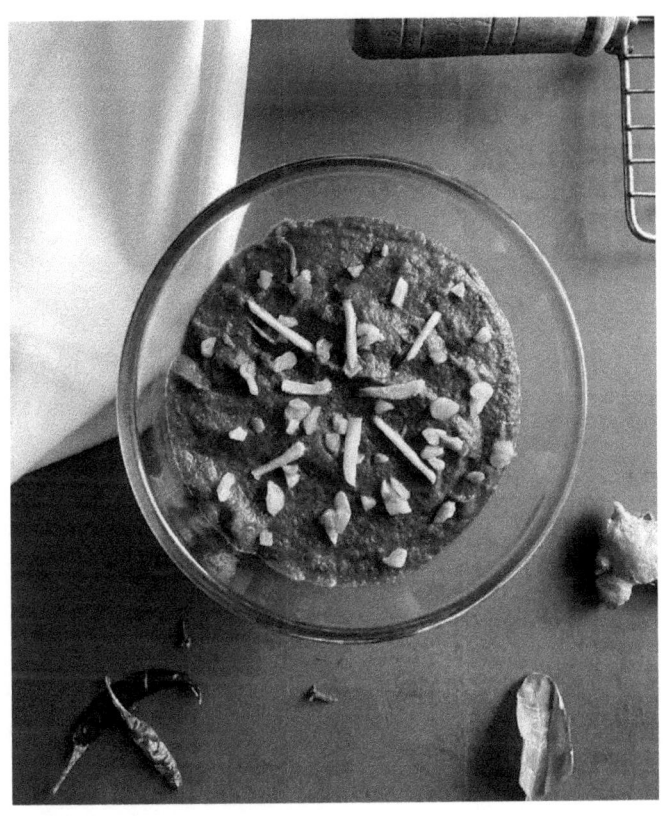

Ingredients

Mustard greens: 175 g	Spinach: 75 g
Lemon juice: 1 tbsp	Maize flour: 2 tbsp
Asafoetida: ¼ tsp	Cumin seeds: ½ tsp
Ginger: 1 inch	Garlic: 5 cloves
Onion: 3	Tomato: 1 medium
Garam masala: 1 tsp	Coriander powder: 1 tsp

Salt: To taste   Water: 250 ml
Rice bran oil: 2 tbsp

For Tampering

Ginger julienne: 1 tbsp   Chopped garlic: 1 tbsp
Asafoetida: A pinch   Red chilli: 1
Butter: 1 tsp

Method

1. Wash the mustard greens and spinach thoroughly. Cut them roughly.

2. Blanch the greens with 50 ml water, salt, and lemon juice for 5 minutes or till the greens are soft.

3. Let it cool down completely. Make a thick puree by grinding the greens with stock and green chilies.

4. Heat oil in a pan. Add asafoetida and cumin. Cook for one minute.

5. Add chopped ginger and garlic. Cook for 2-3 minutes.

6. Add chopped onions. Cover with a lid and cook on low flame for 10 minutes.

7. Add chopped tomatoes and salt (we have added salt during blanching, so add salt accordingly). Cover with a lid and cook on low flame for 10 minutes. Mash the tomatoes with a spatula.

8. Add garam masala and coriander powder. Mix well and cook for 5 minutes.

9. Add maize flour and mix well. Cook for 2 minutes. Add mustard greens and spinach puree and mix well.

10. Add 200 ml water and cook on low flame for 10 minutes. Keep stirring in between, and do not cover the greens. Turn off the flame and add tempering.

For Tempering

1. Heat butter in a pan and add asafoetida, ginger, garlic, and red chili to it. Cook the garlic till it turns brown.

2. Add this tempering to the prepared mustard greens. Immediately cover the greens with a lid. Keep aside for 10 minutes.

3. Enjoy Sarson ka Saag with makki ki roti (maize flour flatbread).

Tips:

1. You can also add other greens like chenopodium, collard, and radish greens with spinach. If using mixed greens, add 125 grams of mustard greens and 125 grams of mixed greens.

2. To retain the bright green color of the greens, do not cover them while blanching.

4. Very little salt is needed in sarson ka saag. You may need half or a quarter of the normal amount. So, add salt according to your taste.

Sign up to La Fonceur Newsletter to receive updates

https://eatsowhat.com/signup

READ OTHER VITAMIN BOOKS

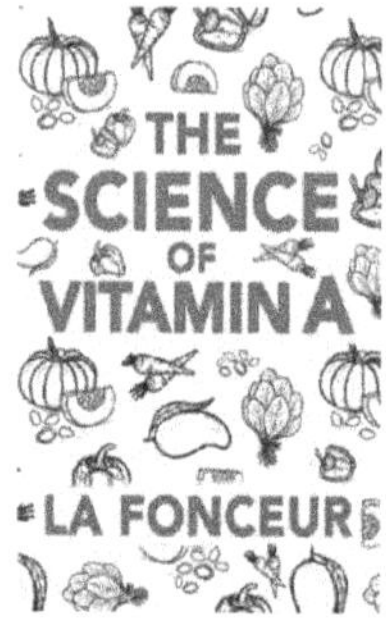

The Science of Vitamin A

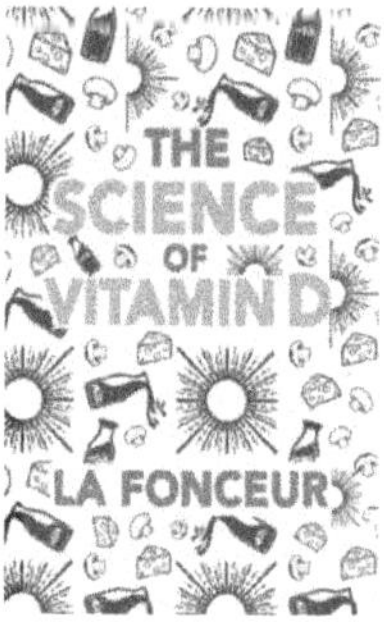

The Science of Vitamin D

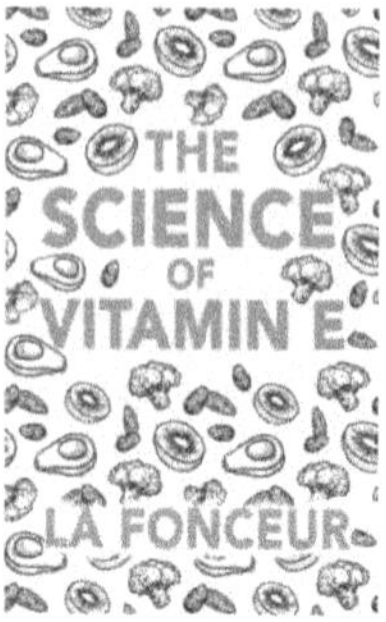

The Science of Vitamin E

REFERENCES

1. Albahrani AA, Greaves RF. Fat-Soluble Vitamins: Clinical Indications and Current Challenges for Chromatographic Measurement. Clin Biochem Rev. 2016 Feb;37(1):27-46.

2. Multivitamin/Mineral Supplements Fact Sheet for Health Professionals, National Institutes of Health.

3. Conly JM, Stein K, Worobetz L, Rutledge-Harding S. The contribution of vitamin K2 (menaquinones) produced by the intestinal microflora to human nutritional requirements for vitamin K. Am J Gastroenterol 1994;89:915-23.

4. Suttie JW. Vitamin K. In: Ross AC, Caballero B, Cousins RJ, Tucker KL, Ziegler TR, eds. Modern Nutrition in Health and Disease. 11th ed. Baltimore, MD: Lippincott Williams & Wilkins; 2014:305-16.

5. Lee S, Choi Y, Jeong HS, Lee J. Effect of cooking methods on the content of vitamins and true retention in selected vegetables. Food Sci Biotechnol. 2017 Dec 12;27(2):333-342.

6. Guylaine, Ferland and James, Sadowski. Vitamin K1 (phylloquinone) content of edible oils: effects of heating and light exposure. Journal of Agricultural and Food Chemistry 1992 40 (10), 1869-1873. DOI: 10.1021/jf00022a028

7. Vitamin K - Health Professional Fact Sheet - National Institues of Health.

8. Widhalm JR, Ducluzeau AL, Basset GJ. Phylloquinone (vitamin K(1)) biosynthesis in plants: two peroxisomal thioesterases of Lactobacillales origin hydrolyze 1,4-dihydroxy-2-naphthoyl-CoA. Plant J. 2012 Jul;71(2):205-15. doi: 10.1111/j.1365-313X.2012.04972.x. Epub 2012 Jun 19.

9. Beulens JW, Booth SL, van den Heuvel EG, Stoecklin E, Baka A, Vermeer C. The role of menaquinones (vitamin K_2) in human health. Br J Nutr. 2013 Oct;110(8):1357-68.

10. Institute of Medicine (US) Panel on Micronutrients. Dietary Reference Intakes for Vitamin A, Vitamin K, Arsenic, Boron, Chromium, Copper, Iodine, Iron, Manganese, Molybdenum, Nickel, Silicon, Vanadium, and Zinc. Washington (DC): National Academies Press (US); 2001. 5, Vitamin K.

11. Shearer MJ, Fu X, Booth SL. Vitamin K nutrition, metabolism, and requirements: current concepts and future research. Adv Nutr 2012;3:182-95.

12. Ronald J. Sokol, Maret G. Traber. Vitamin E and Vitamin K Metabolism. Physiology of the Gastrointestinal Tract (Fourth Edition), 2006.

13. Vitamin K Deficiency Bleeding - Frequently Asked Questions (FAQ's): Vitamin K and the Vitamin K

Shot Given at Birth - Centers for Disease Control and Prevention.

14. Lowenthal J, Birnbaum H. Vitamin K and coumarin anticoagulants: dependence of anticoagulant effect on inhibition of vitamin K transport. Science. 1969 Apr 11;164(3876):181-3.

15. Shearer MJ, Newman P. Metabolism and cell biology of vitamin K. Thromb Haemost. 2008 Oct;100(4):530-47.

16. The Emerging Role of Vitamin K2 Manouchehr Saljoughian, PharmD, PhD Department of Pharmacy, Alta Bates Summit Medical Center, Berkeley, California US Pharm. 2012;37(1):HS-12-HS-14.

17. Clinical and Research Information on Drug-Induced Liver Injury [Internet]. Bethesda (MD): National Institute of Diabetes and Digestive and Kidney Diseases; 2012-. Vitamin K. [Updated 2021 May 27].

18. Fu X, Harshman SG, Shen X, Haytowitz DB, Karl JP, Wolfe BE, Booth SL. Multiple Vitamin K Forms Exist in Dairy Foods. Curr Dev Nutr. 2017 Jun 1;1(6):e000638.

19. Institute of Medicine. Dietary reference intakes for vitamin A, vitamin K, arsenic, boron, chromium, copper, iodine, iron, manganese, molybdenum, nickel, silicon, vanadium, and zinc. Washington, DC: National Academy Press; 2001.

20. Vitamin K Deficiency by Larry E. Johnson, MD, PhD, University of Arkansas for Medical Sciences - MSD Manual Professional Manual.

21. Goto S, Setoguchi S, Matsunaga K, Takata J. Overcoming the Photochemical Problem of Vitamin K in Topical Application. Vitamin K - Recent Topics on the Biology and Chemistry. IntechOpen; 2022.

22. Prothrombin Time Test and INR (PT/INR) - MedlinePlus - National Library of Medicine.

23. Shikdar S, Vashisht R, Bhattacharya PT. International Normalized Ratio (INR) [Updated 2023 May 1] In: StatPearls [Internet]. Treasure Island (FL): StatPearls Publishing; 2023 Jan.

24. Cologne, Germany: Institute for Quality and Efficiency in Health Care (IQWiG); 2006-. What are blood thinners (anti-clotting medication) and how are they used? 2013 Nov 25 [Updated 2017 Oct 5].

25. Sørensen B, Tang M, Larsen OH, Laursen PN, Fenger-Eriksen C, Rea CJ. The role of fibrinogen: a new paradigm in the treatment of coagulopathic bleeding. Thromb Res. 2011;128 Suppl 1:S13-6. doi: 10.1016/S0049-3848(12)70004-X.

26. Celia Rodríguez-Olleros Rodríguez, Manuel Díaz Curiel, "Vitamin K and Bone Health: A Review on the Effects of Vitamin K Deficiency and Supplementation and Effect of Non-Vitamin K Antagonist Oral Anticoagulants on Different Bone

Parameters", Journal of Osteoporosis, vol. 2019, Article ID 2069176, 8 pages, 2019.

27. Maresz K. Proper Calcium Use: Vitamin K2 as a Promoter of Bone and Cardiovascular Health. Integr Med (Encinitas). 2015 Feb;14(1):34-9.

28. Jamie Adams, Joseph Pepping. Vitamin K in Treatment and Prevention of Osteoporosis and Arterial Calcification. American Journal of Health-System Pharmacy. 2005;62(15):1574-1581.

29. Bügel S. Vitamin K and bone health. Proc Nutr Soc. 2003 Nov;62(4):839-43. doi: 10.1079/PNS2003305.

30. Tsugawa, Naoko & Shiraki and Okano, T. Vitamin K status of healthy Japanese women: age-related vitamin K requirement for gamma-carboxylation of osteocalcin. Am J Clin Nutr 83: 380-386. The American journal of clinical nutrition. 83. 380-6. 10.1093/ajcn/83.2.380.

31. Ballegooijen AJ, Pilz S, Tomaschitz A, Grübler MR, Verheyen N. The Synergistic Interplay between Vitamins D and K for Bone and Cardiovascular Health: A Narrative Review. Int J Endocrinol. 2017;2017:7454376.

32. Li Y, Lu X, Yang B, Yasui T, Gao B: Vitamin K1 Inhibition of Renal Crystal Formation through Matrix Gla Protein in the Kidney. Kidney Blood Press Res 2019;44:1392-1403.

33. Girolami A, Ferrari S, Cosi E, Santarossa C, Randi ML. Vitamin K-Dependent Coagulation Factors

That May be Responsible for Both Bleeding and Thrombosis (FII, FVII, and FIX). Clin Appl Thromb Hemost. 2018 Dec;24(9_suppl):42S-47S.

34. Xv F, Chen J, Duan, Li S. Research progress on the anticancer effects of vitamin K2. Oncol Lett. 2018 Jun;15(6):8926-8934.

35. Lu Xin, Ma Panpan, Kong Lingyu, Wang Xi, Wang Yaqi, Jiang Lingling. Vitamin K2 Inhibits Hepatocellular Carcinoma Proliferation by Binding to 17β-Hydroxysteroid Dehydrogenase. Frontiers in Oncology Vol 11 2021.

36. Gary K. Schwartz, Manish A. Shah. Targeting the Cell Cycle: A New Approach to Cancer Therapy. Journal of Clinical Oncology 2005. PG 9408-9421.

37. Office of the Surgeon General (US). Bone Health and Osteoporosis: A Report of the Surgeon General. Rockville (MD): Office of the Surgeon General (US); 2004. 2, The Basics of Bone in Health and Disease.

38. Weber P. Vitamin K and bone health. Nutrition. 2001 Oct;17(10):880-7. doi: 10.1016/0899-9007(01)00709-2. Erratum in: Nutrition 2001 Nov-Dec;17(11-12):1024.

39. Popescu A, German M. Vitamin K2 Holds Promise for Alzheimer's Prevention and Treatment. Nutrients. 2021 Jun 27;13(7):2206. doi: 10.3390/nu13072206.

40. Alisi L, Cao R, De Angelis C, Fiorelli M. The Relationships Between Vitamin K and Cognition: A Review of Current Evidence. Front Neurol. 2019 Mar 19;10:239.

41. Dasgupta S, Ray SK. Diverse Biological Functions of Sphingolipids in the CNS: Ceramide and Sphingosine Regulate Myelination in Developing Brain but Stimulate Demyelination during Pathogenesis of Multiple Sclerosis. J Neurol Psychol. 2017 Dec;5(1):10.13188/2332-3469.1000035.

42. Wishart DS, Feunang YD, Guo AC, Lo EJ, Wilson M. DrugBank 5.0: a major update to the DrugBank database for 2018. Nucleic Acids Res. 2017 Nov 8.

43. Keith DA, Gundberg CM, Japour A, Aronoff J, Alvarez N, Gallop PM. Vitamin K-dependent proteins and anticonvulsant medication. Clin Pharmacol Ther. 1983 Oct;34(4):529-32.

44. Lawson KD, Middleton SJ, Hassall CD. Olestra, a nonabsorbed, noncaloric replacement for dietary fat: a review. Drug Metab Rev. 1997 Aug;29(3):651-703.

45. Food Additives Permitted for Direct Addition to Food for Human Consumption; Olestra. A Rule by the Food and Drug Administration on 08/05/2003.

46. Lee, S., Sung, J., & Lee, J. Analysis of Vitamin K1 in Commonly Consumed Foods in Korea. Journal of the Korean Society of Food Science and Nutrition.

The Korean Society of Food Science and Nutrition. 2015, August 31.

47. Hsiao-Han Lin, Pei-Shan Tsai, Su-Chen Fang, Jen-Fang Liu. Effect of Kiwi Consumption on Sleep Quality in Adults with Sleep Problems. Asia Pacific Journal of Clinical Nutrition. (2011 / 06 / 01), P169 - 174.

48. CFR - Code of Federal Regulations Title 21 - US Food & Drug Administration.

49. Mung beans, mature seeds, sprouted, raw. Food Data Central. US Food & Drug Administration.

50. Peas, green, raw. Food Data Central. US Food & Drug Administration.

51. Traber MG. Vitamin E and K interactions--a 50-year-old problem. Nutr Rev. 2008 Nov;66(11):624-9. doi: 10.1111/j.1753-4887.2008.00123.x.

52. Schwalfenberg GK. Vitamins K1 and K2: The Emerging Group of Vitamins Required for Human Health. J Nutr Metab. 2017;2017:6254836. doi: 10.1155/2017/6254836. Epub 2017 Jun 18.

53. Podszun M, Frank J. Vitamin E-drug interactions: molecular basis and clinical relevance. Nutr Res Rev. 2014 Dec;27(2):215-31. Doi: 10.1017/S0954422414000146. Epub 2014 Sep 16.

54. Kim JM, White RH. Effect of Vitamin E on the anticoagulant response to warfarin. Am J Cardiol.

1996 Mar 1;77(7):545-6. doi: 10.1016/s0002-9149(97)89357-5.

55. Fan Y, Adam TJ, McEwan R, Pakhomov SV, Melton GB, Zhang R. Detecting Signals of Interactions Between Warfarin and Dietary Supplements in Electronic Health Records. Stud Health Technol Inform. 2017;245:370-374.

56. Lanham-New SA. Importance of calcium, vitamin D and vitamin K for osteoporosis prevention and treatment. Proc Nutr Soc. 2008 May;67(2):163-76. doi: 10.1017/S0029665108007003.

57. Saboori S, Djalali M, Nematipour E, Ramezani A. Various Effects of Omega 3 and Omega 3 Plus Vitamin E Supplementations on Serum Glucose Level and Insulin Resistance in Patients with Coronary Artery Disease. Iran J Public Health. 2016 Nov;45(11):1465-1472.

58. M. Sepidarkish, M. Morvaridzadeh, J. Heshmati. Effect of omega-3 fatty acid and vitamin E Co-Supplementation on lipid profile: a systematic review and meta-analysis. Diabetes Metab. Syndr. Clin. Res. Rev., 13 (2019), pp. 1649-1656

59. Lu, T.; Shen, Y.; Wang, J.H.; Xie, H.K.; Wang, Y.F.; Zhao, Q.; Zhou, D.-Y.; Shahidi, F. Improving oxidative stability of flaxseed oil with a mixture of antioxidants. J. Food Proc. Preserv. 2020, 44, e14355.

60. Floros S, Toskas A, Vareltzis P. Bioaccessibility, Oxidative Stability of Omega-3 Fatty Acids in Supplements, Sardines and Enriched Eggs Studied Using a Static In Vitro Gastrointestinal Model. Molecules. 2022 Jan 9;27(2):415. doi: 10.3390/molecules27020415.

61. Bischoff-Ferrari HA, Willett WC, Manson JE, Gaengler S. Combined Vitamin D, Omega-3 Fatty Acids, a Simple Home Exercise Program May Reduce Cancer Risk Among Active Adults Aged 70 and Older: A Randomized Clinical Trial. Front Aging. 2022 Apr 25;3:852643. doi: 10.3389/fragi.2022.852643.

62. Maresz K. Proper Calcium Use: Vitamin K2 as a Promoter of Bone and Cardiovascular Health. Integr Med (Encinitas). 2015 Feb;14(1):34-9.

63. Hu, L., Li, D. et al. The combined effect of vitamin K and calcium on bone mineral density in humans: analysis of randomized controlled trials. J Orthop Surg Res 16, 592 (2021). https://doi.org/10.1186/s13018-021-02728-4

64. Maresz K. Proper Calcium Use: Vitamin K2 as a Promoter of Bone and Cardiovascular Health. Integr Med (Encinitas). 2015 Feb;14(1):34-9.

ABOUT THE AUTHOR

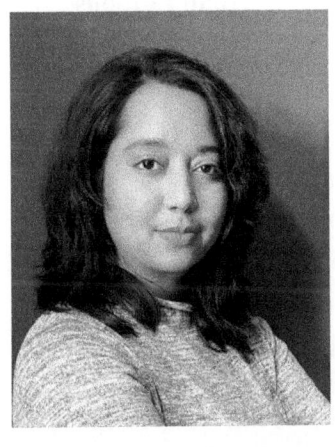

With a Master's Degree in Pharmacy, the author La Fonceur is a Research Scientist and Registered Pharmacist. She specialized in Pharmaceutical Technology and worked as a research scientist in the pharmaceutical research and development department. She is a health blogger and a dance artist. Her previous books include Eat to Prevent and Control Disease, Secret of Healthy Hair, and Eat So What! series. Being a research scientist, she has worked closely with drugs and based on her experience, she believes that one can prevent most of the diseases with nutritious vegetarian foods and a healthy lifestyle.

READ MORE FROM LA FONCEUR

English Editions	**Hindi Editions**

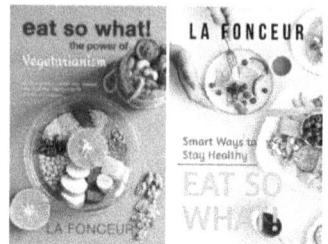
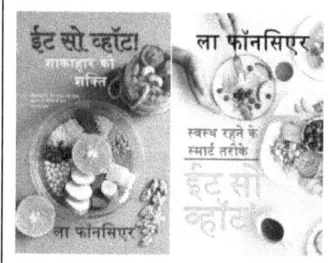

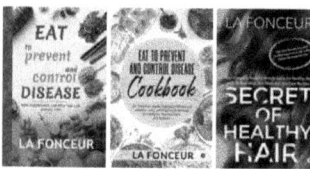
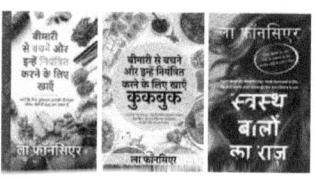

CONNECT WITH LA FONCEUR

Instagram: @la_fonceur | @eatsowhat

Facebook: LaFonceur | eatsowhatblog

Twitter: @la_fonceur

Follow on Bookbub: @eatsowhat

Sign up to get exclusive offers on La Fonceur books:

Blog: https://www.eatsowhat.com/

Website: https://www.lafonceur.com/

www.ingramcontent.com/pod-product-compliance
Ingram Content Group UK Ltd.
Pitfield, Milton Keynes, MK11 3LW, UK
UKHW021021100325
455944UK00010B/376

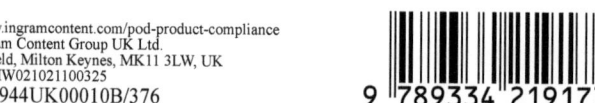